D1644830

Trail Guide
to the Body's
QUICK REFERENCE TO
Stretch & Strengthen

Andrew Biel, LMP

Illustrations by
Robin Dorn, LMP

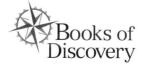

Books of
Discovery

First Edition

Published by Books of Discovery
2539 Spruce St., Boulder, CO 80302 USA
www.booksofdiscovery.com
800.775.9227

Designed by Jessica Xavier of Planet X Design

Printed by Kromar Printing in Winnipeg, Canada

Library of Congress Cataloging-in-Publication Data

Biel, Andrew R.
Trail Guide to the Body's Quick Reference to Stretch & Strengthen

Includes index.

ISBN: 978-0-9829786-1-0
Library of Congress Control Number: 2011919889

15 14 13 12 11 10 9 8 7 6 5 4 3 2 1

Disclaimer

*This book does not offer medical advice to the reader and is not intended as
a replacement for appropriate health care and treatment. For such advice,
readers should consult a licensed physician. Proper exercise programs should
be supervised by a personal trainer or physician and the exercises included in
this text are not designed to replace prescribed rehabilitative exercises.*

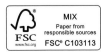

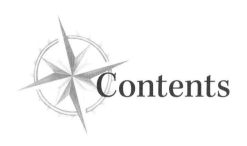

Contents

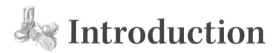 # Introduction

Our flagship text, *Trail Guide to the Body: A hands-on guide to locating muscles, bones and more* covers the subject of palpatory anatomy. This booklet is designed to present two neighboring subjects of palpation—stretching and strengthening. Each of these topics could fill several books. The intent of this short text is to introduce these fundamental subjects to students and practitioners of manual therapy.

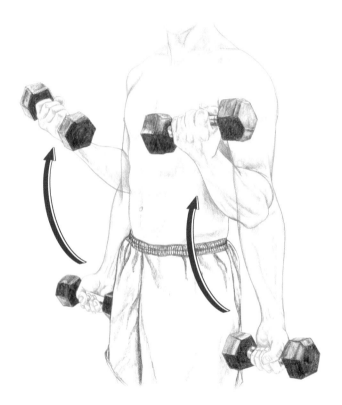

   Please note that some of the stretching and strengthening images include the rendering of a specific muscle. This has been inserted when visually possible and to show how the muscle is involved in an exercise. It is not meant to indicate that only one muscle is participating.

   We've kept the exercises as simple as possible. A short list of equipment includes light dumbbells, a long strip of elastic such as a Thera-band and a floor mat or yoga mat. Some of the exercises involve the use of pulleys, which may require access to a local gym.

Stretching

Although the research on the benefits of stretching shows mixed results, the primary advantage of stretching is to improve flexibility. Being more flexible may improve athletic performance and decrease the risk of injury to muscles and surrounding tissues by allowing joints to move through their full range of motion.

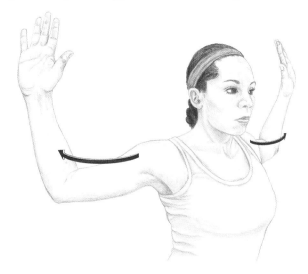

There's another reason to stretch——it feels good (if you have doubts, ask a cat). Take, for example, our most primal form of stretching, the yawn. Aside from providing a gentle expansion of the mouth, face and diaphragm, this mysterious gesture sends a relaxing message throughout the entire nervous system. Personally, my favorite time to stretch is before I climb into bed. A few minutes of gentle, broad movement makes the day's tension drop off.

There are many different stretching techniques. Some yoga styles, Pilates and PNF (proprioceptive neuromuscular facilitation), for example, all offer various ways to stretch (and strengthen). This manual presents static stretches. These are movements/positions that passively stretch a muscle (or area of the body) to a point of mild discomfort for 30 to 60 seconds. They are straightforward, very effective and relatively safe. In other words, they're great for beginners.

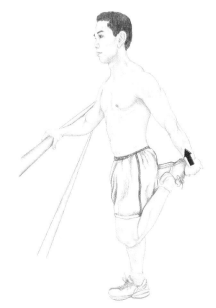

Here are a few guidelines to get the most out of your stretching:

- Stretching can be done before and after exercise, but before you stretch, warm up with light walking, easy jogging or biking for 5 to 10 minutes.

- Stretch slowly and stay relaxed. Your hamstrings (or any other muscle) won't take kindly to rapid, aggressive stretching. Take it easy and remember that you're stretching live tissue, not Saran Wrap over a bulging bowl of fruit.

- Hold each stretch for 30 to 60 seconds.

- Listen to your body. When you're wondering how far you should stretch your pectorals, check in with them. They'll let you know.

- Avoid bouncing or stretching to the point of pain. This will actually sabotage your intention by causing a muscle to "pull."

- Breathe. Slow, deep breaths can assist in deepening the stretch.

- To maintain the flexibility you have gained, consider stretching at least three times a week.

- Try to reserve 10 to 20 minutes for each stretching session.

- With that said, stretching doesn't have to be a formal event. Short, focused stretching sessions at your desk or while waiting for a bus can be quite beneficial as well.

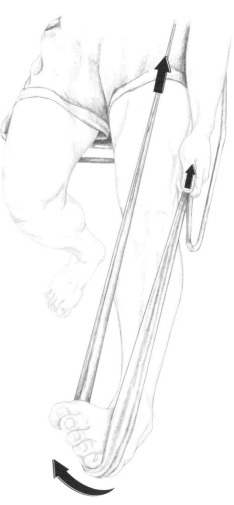

Strengthening

The benefits of strengthening exercises include reducing the risk of injury; increasing balance, stability and flexibility and—of course—keeping your body strong. As with stretching, there are many ways to strengthen your muscles, such as general exercise or athletic activities. For this manual, weight training will be the type of strength techniques described. All of these exercises are clear cut, isolated to specific muscles and—if performed properly—challenging, but not difficult. Again, good for beginners.

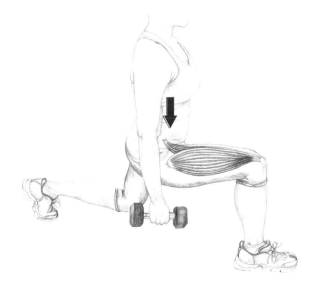

Here are a few basic principles to follow when weight training:

- Begin each session by doing 10 minutes of light cardio exercise on a stationary bike or treadmill. This will help warm up your muscles for lifting.

- Choose an exercise for each muscle group and do 1–2 sets of 8–15 repetitions for each exercise.

- How much weight should you use? Optimally, an amount that you can lift 8–15 times without excessive stress. Of course, the point of weight training is to stress muscles, but your lifting should be smooth and not compromise your posture or breathing.

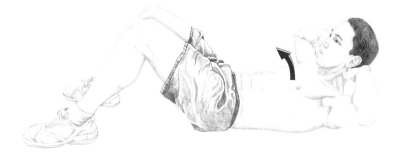

- Lift and lower the weight slowly and gracefully, following your breath as you go. Also, try not to use momentum to lift the weight. If you have to swing the weight up, you're using too much weight.

- Lift the weight through the joint's entire range of motion. An elbow curl that only involves 30 percent of potential range won't be as effective as the full movement.

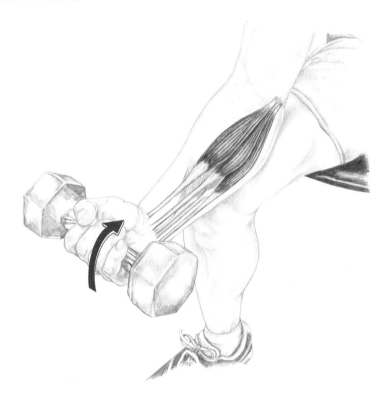

- Be aware of your body position and posture. For example, are your hips, shoulders and head in alignment? Are your feet stable? Are your pelvis and lumbar spine balanced front to back?

- Remember that your rest days are just as important as your workout days. Consider weight training 2 to 3 times a week with at least one day off between sessions.

- Remember that you're just trying to strengthen your muscles, not to become Mr. or Ms. Universe. (Well, maybe you are, who knows?) Relax and enjoy.

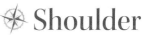

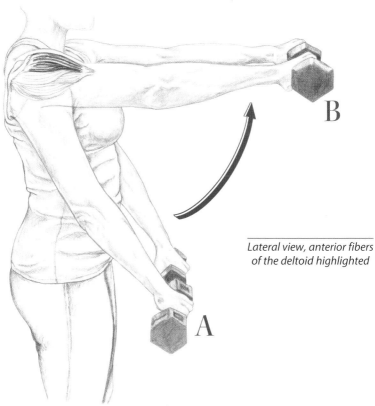

Lateral view, anterior fibers of the deltoid highlighted

Shoulder Flexors – Strengthen

1) Standing, with a dumbbell in each hand and your forearms pronated (A). Keeping your elbows extended, flex your shoulders to 90 degrees (B).

2) Return to the starting position.

✳ Shoulder

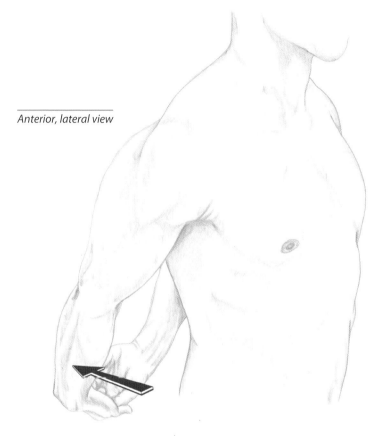

Anterior, lateral view

Shoulder Flexors – Stretch

1) Standing. Interlace your fingers behind your back with your palms up. (Note how this hand position is different from the stretch for the elbow flexors on p. 38.)

2) Keeping your elbows extended, begin to extend your shoulders. While stretching, try to maintain an erect torso to prevent the shoulders from rolling forward.

3) Take several deep breaths and then slowly return to the starting position.

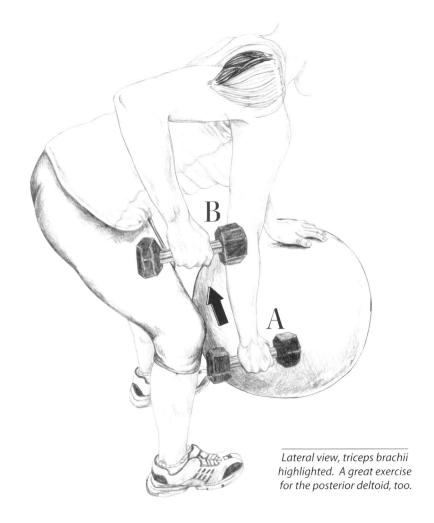

Lateral view, triceps brachii highlighted. A great exercise for the posterior deltoid, too.

Shoulder Extensors – Strengthen

Variation 1

1) Standing, with a big ball (or chair) in front of you and a dumbbell in your right hand. Flex your hips and place your left hand on the ball. Now you are in position (A).

2) As you extend your shoulder, raise your elbow toward the ceiling (but allow your elbow to flex). (B)

3) Raise the elbow only to a comfortable point and then return to the starting position.

✦ Shoulder

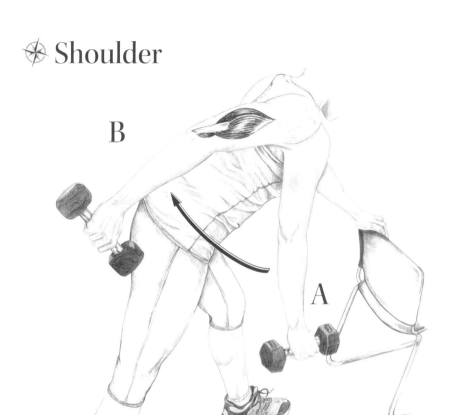

B

A

Lateral view, posterior fibers of deltoid highlighted. A great exercise for the triceps brachii, too.

Shoulder Extensors – Strengthen

Variation 2 *By engaging the posterior fibers of the deltoid, this exercise also applies to horizontal abduction of the shoulder.*

1) Standing, with a dumbbell in your right hand. Begin with your left foot forward and your right foot back.

2) Lean forward and stabilize yourself on a chair (or big ball) with your left hand. Begin with your right arm hanging toward the floor. Now you are in position (A).

3) Keep your right elbow extended as you extend your shoulder (B). Raise the arm only to a comfortable point and then return to the starting position.

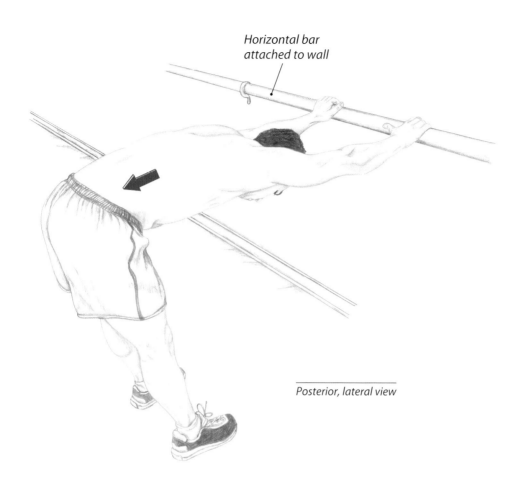

Horizontal bar
attached to wall

Posterior, lateral view

Shoulder Extensors – Stretch

1) Stand in front of a horizontal bar (or table or back of a chair) that is waist high. Hold onto the bar for support and walk your feet back, flexing at the hips.

2) Now, with your shoulders in a flexed position, you can take several deep breaths and then return to the starting position (standing upright).

3) To accentuate the stretch, gently lean your weight back–away from the bar—onto your heels.

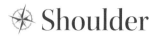 Shoulder

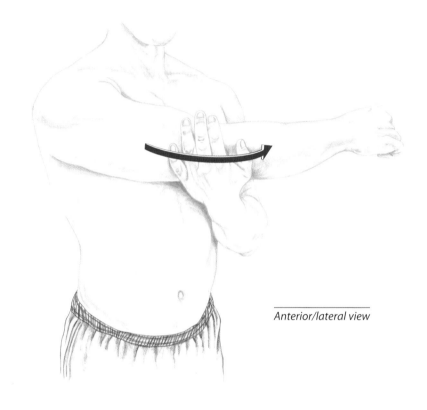

Anterior/lateral view

Shoulder Horizontal Abductors – Stretch

1) Standing. Horizontally adduct your right shoulder (bringing it in front of your chest).

2) For support, reach your left hand under your right elbow to assist with pulling the elbow across the upper chest. Be careful not to rotate your torso (thus reducing the potential stretch).

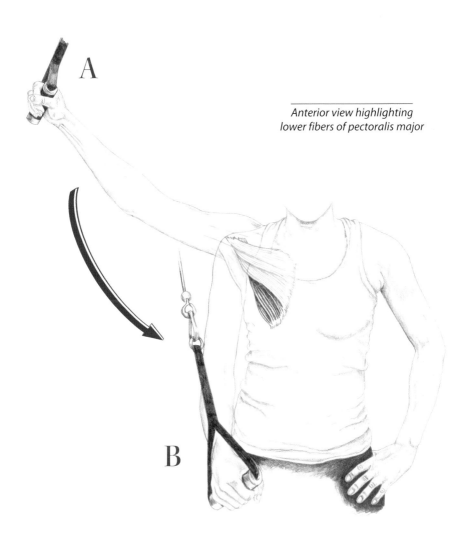

A

*Anterior view highlighting
lower fibers of pectoralis major*

B

Shoulder Horizontal Adductors – Strengthen

Variation 1 – Downward angle

1) Standing, with a cable handle in your right hand. The source of the cable resistance is from the side and above your head. Begin with your shoulder abducted (hand up over your head–A).

2) Slowly horizontally adduct your shoulder at a downward angle, bringing the handle down and across the front of your torso (B).

3) Following the same path, slowly return the shoulder to the starting position.

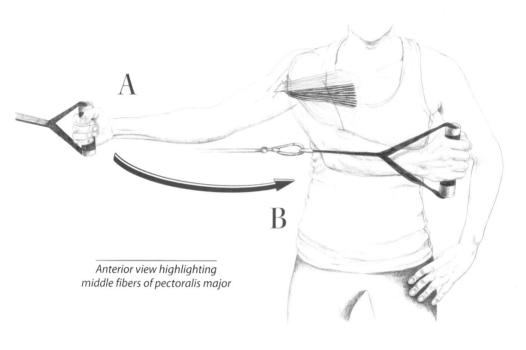

A

B

*Anterior view highlighting
middle fibers of pectoralis major*

Shoulder Horizontal Adductors – Strengthen

Variation 2 – Horizontal angle

1) Standing, with the cable handle in your right hand. The source of the cable resistance is from the side and at shoulder level.

2) Begin with your shoulder partially abducted (hand at shoulder level–A). Slowly horizontally adduct your shoulder, bringing the handle across the front of your chest (B).

3) Following the same path, slowly return the shoulder to the starting position.

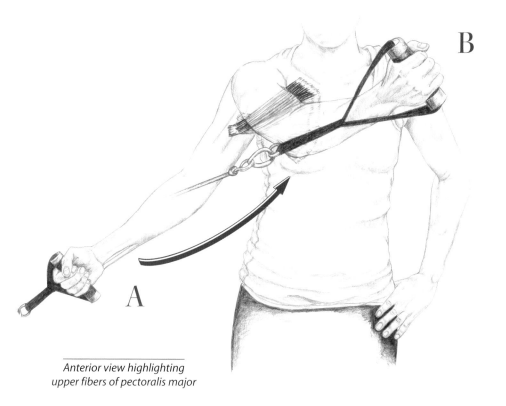

*Anterior view highlighting
upper fibers of pectoralis major*

Shoulder Horizontal Adductors – Strengthen

Variation 3 – Upward angle

1) Standing, with the cable handle in your right hand. The source of the cable resistance is from the side and at floor level.

2) Begin with your shoulder slightly abducted (hand at hip level–A). Slowly horizontally adduct and flex your shoulder, bringing the handle up and across the front of your torso (B).

3) Following the same path, slowly return the shoulder to the starting position.

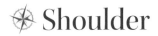

Shoulder

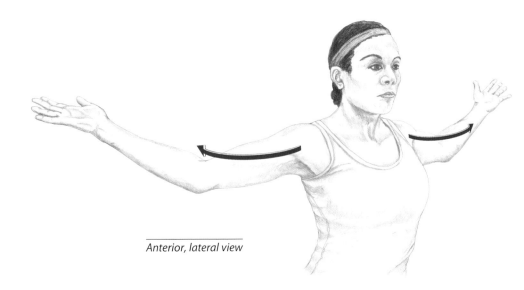

Anterior, lateral view

Shoulder Horizontal Adductors – Stretch

Variation 1 – Elbows extended

1) Standing. Begin with both arms straight out in front of you.
2) Keeping your elbows extended and your palms up, horizontally abduct your shoulders. A few deep breaths that expand the rib cage can accentuate the stretch.

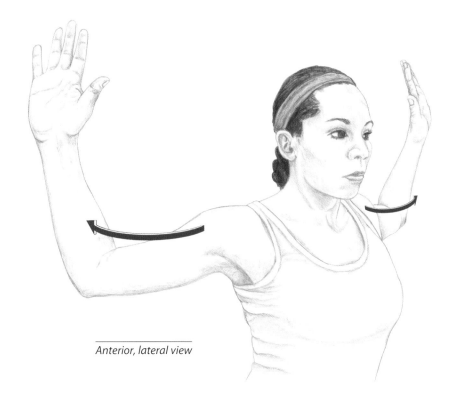

Anterior, lateral view

Shoulder Horizontal Adductors – Stretch

Variation 2 – Elbows flexed

1) Standing. Begin with both arms straight out in front of you.

2) Bend the elbows to 90 degrees and then horizontally abduct your shoulders. Your palms should be facing straight ahead. A few deep breaths that expand the rib cage can accentuate the stretch.

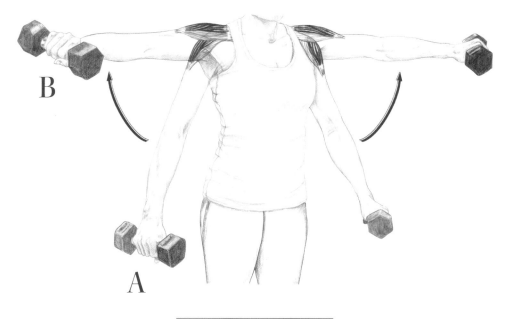

*Anterior, lateral view highlighting
middle fibers of deltoid*

Shoulder Abductors – Strengthen

1) Standing, with a dumbbell in each hand. Forearms can be pronated or in neutral. Begin with your arms at your sides (A).

2) Keeping your elbows in an extended position, abduct your shoulders (B). Raise the arms only to a comfortable height and then return to the starting position.

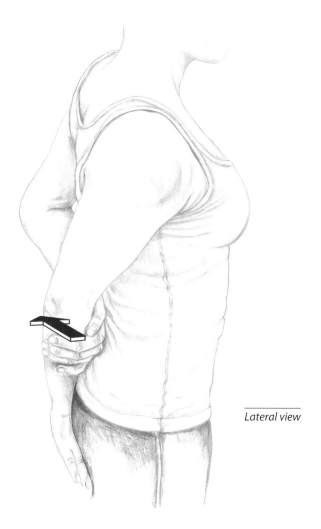

Lateral view

Shoulder Abductors – Stretch

1) Standing. Adduct your right shoulder so that your arm is behind your back.

2) Reach your left hand behind your back and grasp your right elbow. Now you are in position for the stretch.

3) Use your left hand to passively adduct your right shoulder. Be sure that the right arm remains alongside the torso and that the right shoulder does not elevate.

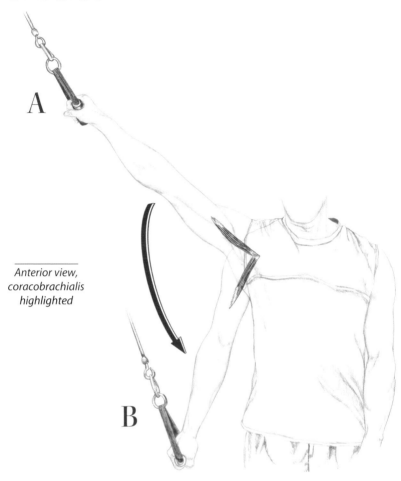

Anterior view, coracobrachialis highlighted

Shoulder Adductors – Strengthen

Variation 1 – Pulley

1) Standing, with a cable handle in your right hand. The source of the cable resistance is from the side and above your head.

2) Begin with your shoulder in an abducted position (hand up over your head) and your forearm pronated (A).

3) Slowly horizontally adduct your shoulder, bringing the handle down to the side of your torso (B). Then slowly return the arm to the starting position.

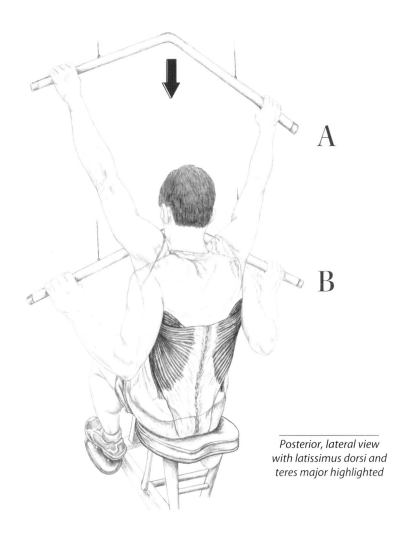

A

B

Posterior, lateral view
with latissimus dorsi and
teres major highlighted

Shoulder Adductors – Strengthen

Variation 2 – Pull-down machine

1) Instead of a "pull-up," this is a "pull-down." Position yourself in the pull-down machine and grasp the bar over your head.

2) Set both hands wider than your shoulders with your forearms in a pronated position (A).

3) As you exhale, slowly adduct your shoulders and bring the bar down to the level of your clavicles (B). Slowly return to the starting position.

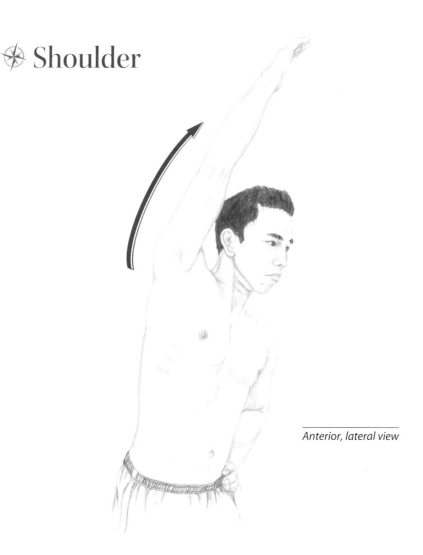

Anterior, lateral view

Shoulder Adductors – Stretch

1) Standing. Set your left hand on your hip and abduct your right shoulder so that your arm is alongside your head.

2) As you reach your fingers up and toward the other side of your body, take some slow deep breaths.

3) Laterally flexing the torso can increase the stretch's range.

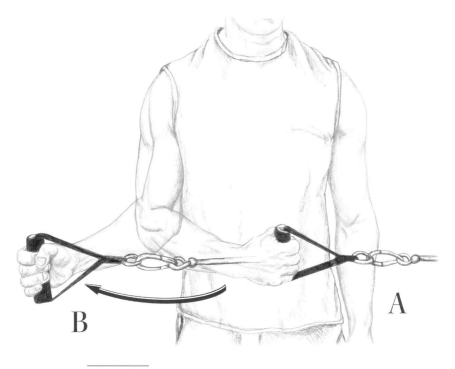

B

A

Anterior view

Shoulder Lateral Rotators – Strengthen

1) Standing, with a cable handle in your right hand. The source of the cable resistance is from your left side and at hip level.

2) Begin with your shoulder internally rotated and the elbow flexed at 90 degrees (A).

3) Keep your elbow next to your torso as you slowly bring the handle horizontally away from your torso (externally rotating the shoulder–B). Then slowly return the shoulder to the starting position.

✳ Shoulder

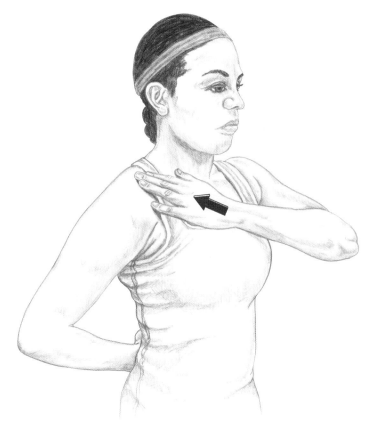

Anterior, lateral view

Shoulder Lateral Rotators – Stretch

1) Standing. Put your right hand in the small of your back and place your left hand on the front of your right shoulder.

2) To begin the stretch (and further rotate the shoulder internally), very gently press your right elbow anteriorly while your left hand stabilizes the right shoulder from rolling forward.

3) Raising the chest and taking some deep breaths can accentuate the stretch.

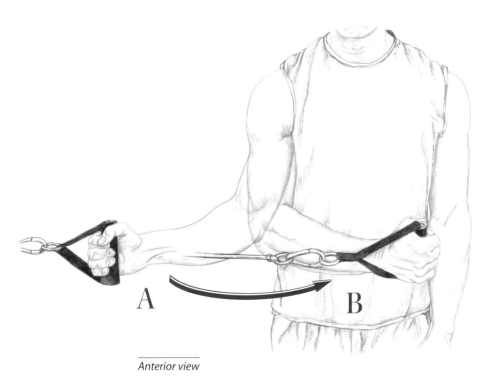

Anterior view

Shoulder Medial Rotators – Strengthen

1) Standing, with a cable handle in your right hand. The source of the cable resistance is from your right side and at hip level.

2) Begin with your shoulder externally rotated and the elbow flexed at 90 degrees (A). Keep your elbow next to your torso as you slowly bring the handle horizontally across your front (internally rotating the shoulder–B).

3) Slowly return the shoulder to the starting position.

✳ Shoulder

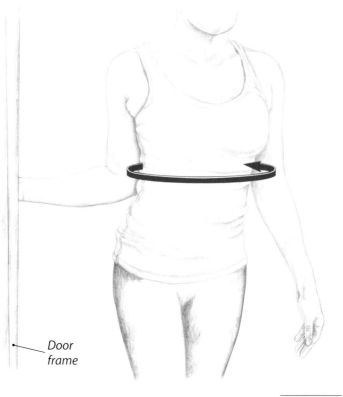

Door frame

Anterior view

Shoulder Medial Rotators – Stretch

1) Standing in a doorway, flex your right elbow to 90 degrees and externally rotate your shoulder with your fingers hooked behind the door frame.

2) Keeping your elbow next to your side, slowly rotate your torso to the left (thus further externally rotating the shoulder).

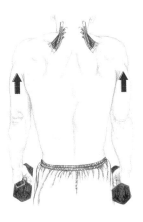

*Posterior view with
levator scapula
highlighted*

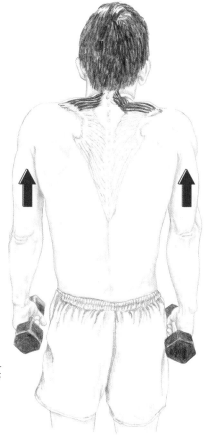

*Posterior view with upper fibers
of trapezius highlighted*

Scapula Elevators – Strengthen

1) Standing, with a dumbbell in each hand.
2) Slowly elevate your scapulae and then return to the starting position.

✳ Scapula

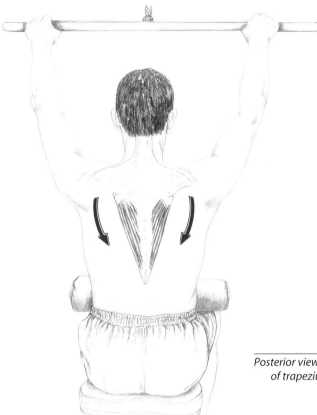

*Posterior view with lower fibers
of trapezius highlighted*

Scapula Depressors – Strengthen

This exercise involves little movement but will still engage the lower fibers of the trapezius.

1) Begin seated in a "pull-down" machine. Grasp the bar over your head and position both hands wider than your shoulders.

2) Your forearms should be pronated. Keeping your elbows extended, slowly depress your scapulae down toward your hips. Again, this will be a small movement.

3) Slowly return to the starting position.

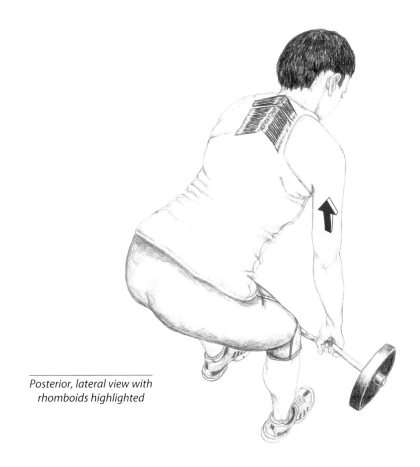

Posterior, lateral view with rhomboids highlighted

Scapula Adductors – Strengthen

Variation 1 *Like the depressor exercise on page 30, this involves a small "shrug" of the shoulders.*

1) Standing, with a long bar (or dumbbells) in your hands. Lean your torso forward at 45 degrees with your arms hanging toward the floor.

2) Keeping your elbows extended, slowly adduct your scapulae by raising your shoulders toward the ceiling.

3) Slowly return to the starting position.

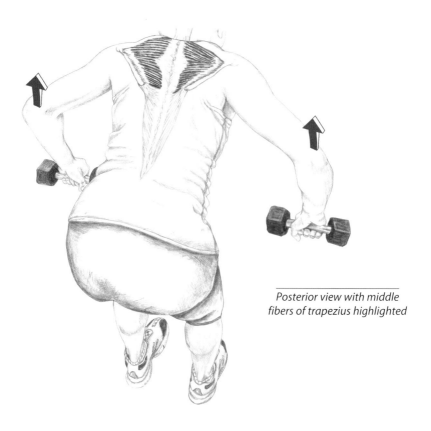

Posterior view with middle fibers of trapezius highlighted

Scapula Adductors – Strengthen

Variation 2

1) Standing, with a dumbbell in each hand. Flex your hips so your torso is leaning forward at 45 degrees and your arms are hanging toward the floor. Now you are in position.

2) Raise your elbows up and to the outside, horizontally abducting your shoulders (the scapulae will adduct as well).

3) Return your elbows to the starting position.

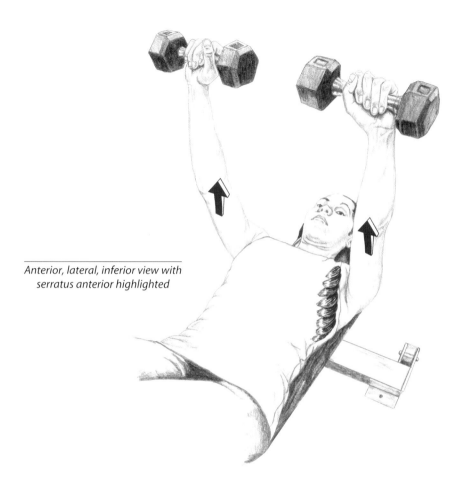

Anterior, lateral, inferior view with
serratus anterior highlighted

Scapula Abductors – Strengthen

Variation 1 *This is a good exercise to target the serratus anterior.*

1) Lie supine on a slender bench with a dumbbell in each hand. Raise your arms so the weights are toward the ceiling.

2) Holding your arms there, let your scapulae shift toward the floor (adducting the scapulae). Now you are ready for the exercise.

3) Keeping your arms in place, slowly shrug your scapulae up toward the ceiling (abduction). The actual movement of the scapulae will be small.

4) Allow the scapulae to shift back toward the floor to the starting position.

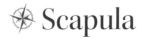

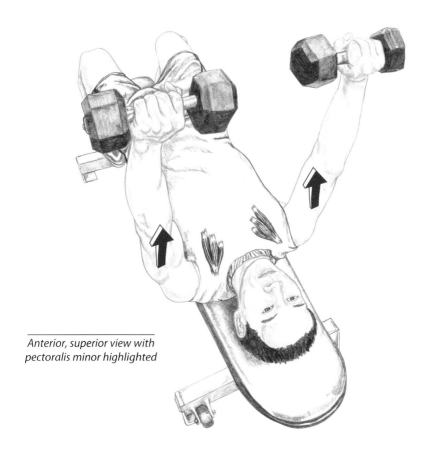

Anterior, superior view with pectoralis minor highlighted

Scapula Abductors – Strengthen

Variation 2 *This is a good exercise to target the pectoralis minor.*

1) Lie supine on a slender bench (hips higher than your head) with a dumbbell in each hand. Raise your arms so the weights are toward the ceiling.

2) Holding your arms there, let your scapulae shift toward the floor (adducting the scapulae). Now you are ready for the exercise.

3) Keeping your arms in place, slowly shrug your scapulae up toward the ceiling (abduction). The actual movement of the scapulae will be small.

4) Allow the scapulae to shift toward the floor to the starting position.

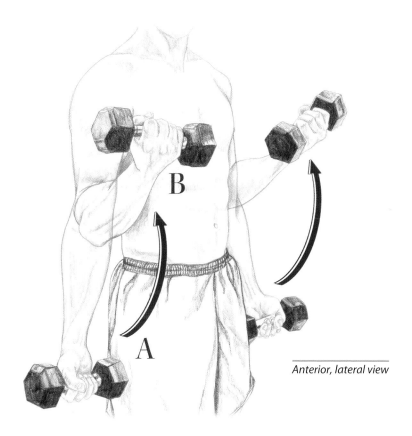

Anterior, lateral view

Elbow Flexors – Strengthen

Variation 1 *A good exercise for the biceps brachii.*

1) Standing, with a dumbbell in each hand and your forearms supinated (A).
2) Keep your shoulders in place and flex your elbows. Raise the dumbbells just past 90 degrees (B) and then slowly return to the starting position.

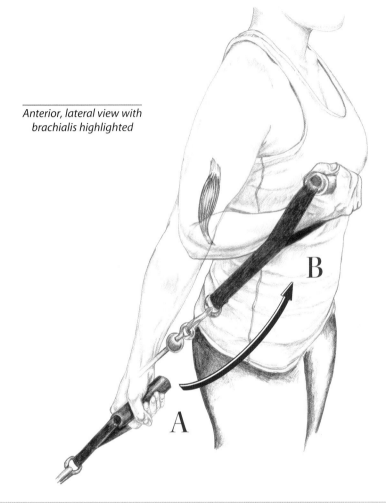

Anterior, lateral view with brachialis highlighted

Elbow Flexors – Strengthen

Variation 2 *A good exercise for the brachialis.*

1) Standing, with cable handle in right hand. The source of the cable resistance is behind you and at floor level.

2) Begin with your arm down at your side, elbow extended and forearm pronated (A). Flex your elbow and raise the handle just past 90 degrees (B). Then slowly return to the starting position.

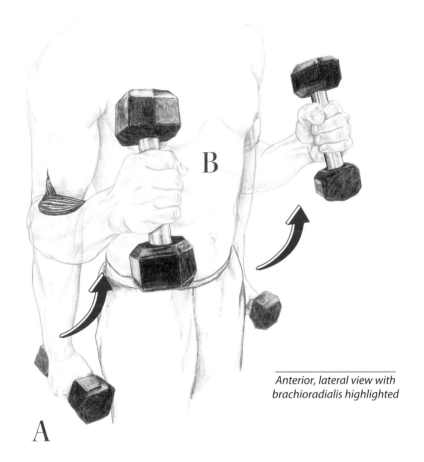

Anterior, lateral view with brachioradialis highlighted

B

A

Elbow Flexors – Strengthen

Variation 3 *A good exercise for the brachioradialis.*

1) Standing, with a dumbbell in each hand and your forearms in a neutral position (A).

2) Keep your shoulders in place and flex your elbows. Raise the dumbbells just past 90 degrees (B) and then slowly return to the starting position.

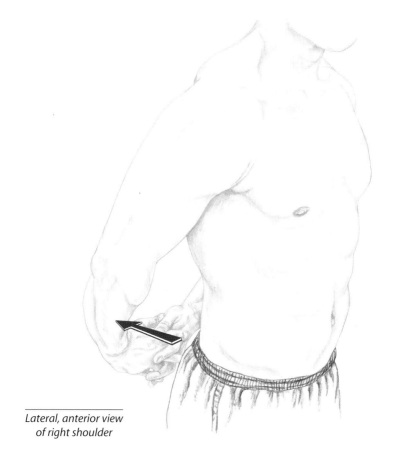

*Lateral, anterior view
of right shoulder*

Elbow Flexors – Stretch

1) Standing. Interlace your fingers behind your back with your palms down. (Note how this hand position is different from the stretch for the shoulder flexors on p. 10.)

2) Keeping your elbows extended, begin to extend your shoulders. Hold the stretch for several breaths and then release.

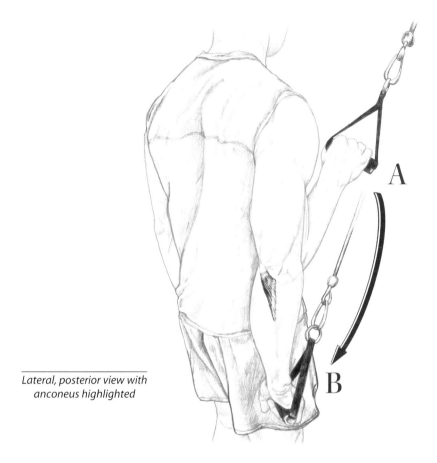

Lateral, posterior view with anconeus highlighted

Elbow Extensors – Strengthen

Variation 1 – *A great exercise for the triceps brachii, as well.*

1) Standing, with cable handle in right hand. The source of the cable resistance is in front of you and above your head.

2) Begin with your elbow fully flexed and your forearm pronated (A). Keeping your elbow against your side, bring the handle down to the side of your hip (extending your elbow–B).

3) Slowly return to the starting position.

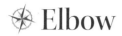

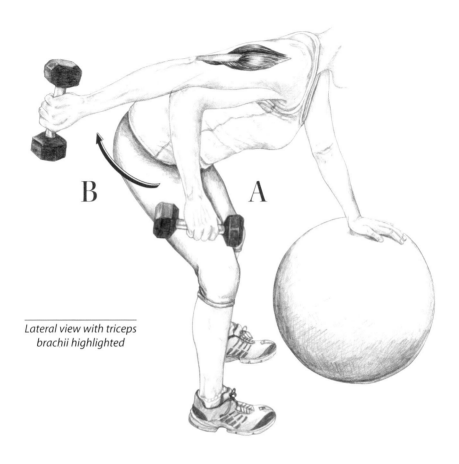

Lateral view with triceps brachii highlighted

Elbow Extensors – Strengthen

Variation 2

1) Standing, with a big ball in front of you and a dumbbell in your right hand. Flex your torso and rest your left hand on the ball.

2) Begin with your right elbow flexed and your forearm in neutral (A). Then extend your elbow fully, lifting the dumbbell (B).

3) Slowly return to the starting position.

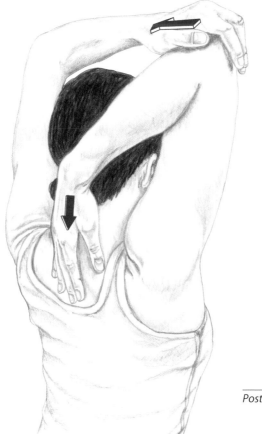

Posterior, lateral view

Elbow Extensors – Stretch

1) Standing. Reach your hand overhead and then fully flex your right elbow. (Your hand will be positioned between your scapulae.)

2) Use your left hand to gently bring the right elbow posteriorly and toward the left.

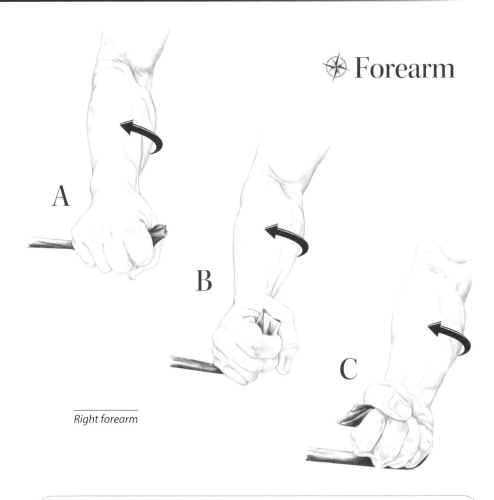

Right forearm

Forearm Supinators – Strengthen

1) Standing or seated. Tie the end of an elastic strap around a doorknob (or other stationary item) to your right. Hold the end of the strap in your right hand and flex your elbow to 90 degrees.

2) Begin with your forearm in a pronated position (A) and then slowly supinate against the resistance of the strap (B).

3) When your forearm is fully supinated (C), slowly return the forearm to a pronated position.

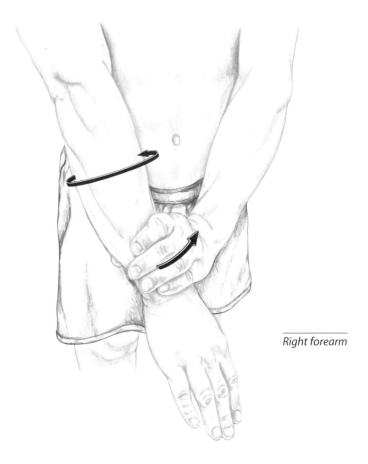

Right forearm

Forearm Supinators – Stretch

1) Standing. Begin with your right elbow extended and your forearm pronated.

2) Grasp the distal end of your right forearm with your left hand (palm down) and then further pronate your forearm.

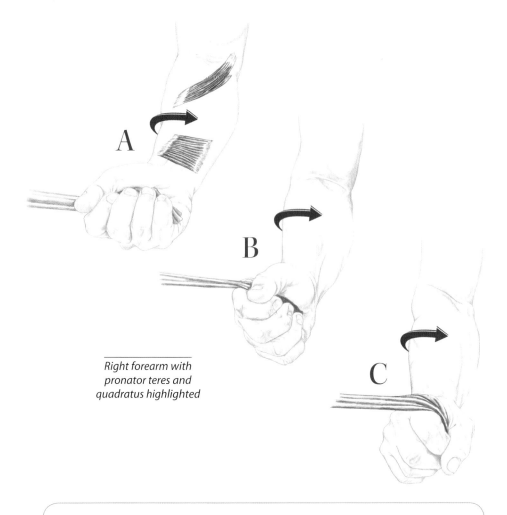

A

B

C

*Right forearm with
pronator teres and
quadratus highlighted*

Forearm Pronators – Strengthen

1) Standing or seated. Tie the end of an elastic strap around a doorknob (or other stationary item) to your right. Hold the strap in your right hand and flex your elbow to 90 degrees.

2) Begin with your forearm in a supinated position (A) and then slowly pronate against the resistance of the strap (B).

3) When your forearm is fully pronated (C), slowly return the forearm to a supinated position.

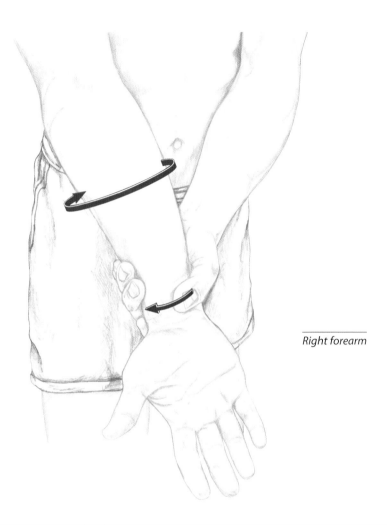

Right forearm

Forearm Pronators – Stretch

1) Standing. Begin with your right elbow extended and your forearm supinated.

2) Grasp the distal end of your right forearm with your left hand (palm up) and further supinate your forearm. Be sure your shoulder does not externally rotate, thus minimizing the stretch.

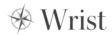

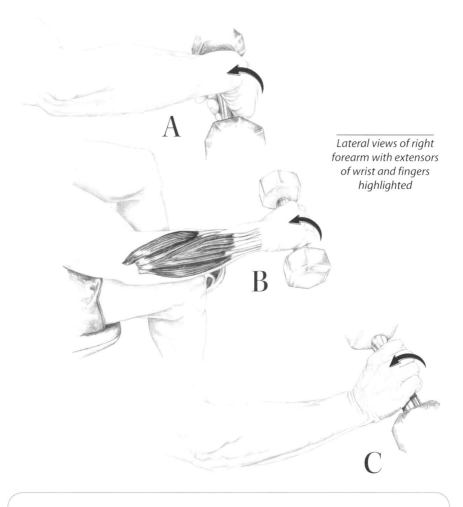

A

Lateral views of right forearm with extensors of wrist and fingers highlighted

B

C

Wrist Extensors – Strengthen

1) Seated, with a dumbbell in your right hand. Rest your right forearm on your thigh so the dumbbell is out over your knee.

2) With your forearm pronated and the wrist in a flexed position (A), begin the exercise by slowly extending your wrist (B).

3) When the wrist is fully extended (C), return to the starting position.

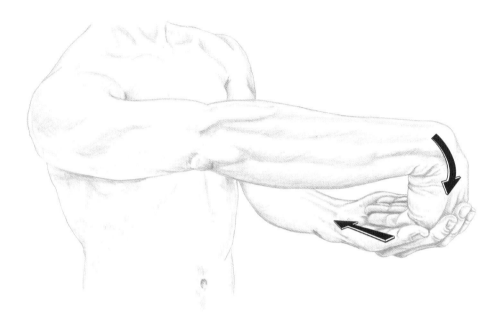

Right forearm and hand

Wrist Extensors – Stretch

1) Standing. Extend your right elbow and make a soft fist with your right hand.
2) As you slowly curl (flex) your wrist, set your left hand on the back of your right hand to assist the stretch.

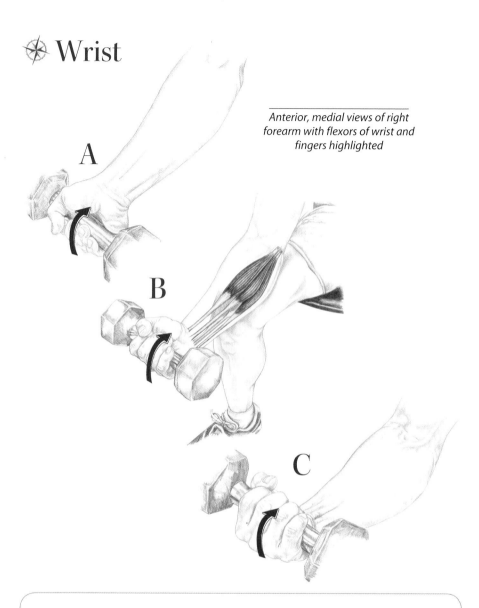

Anterior, medial views of right forearm with flexors of wrist and fingers highlighted

A

B

C

Wrist Flexors – Strengthen

1) Seated, with a dumbbell in your right hand. Rest your right forearm on your thigh so the dumbbell hangs out over your knee.

2) With your forearm supinated and the wrist in extension (A), begin the exercise by slowly flexing your wrist (B).

3) When the wrist is fully flexed (C), return to the starting position.

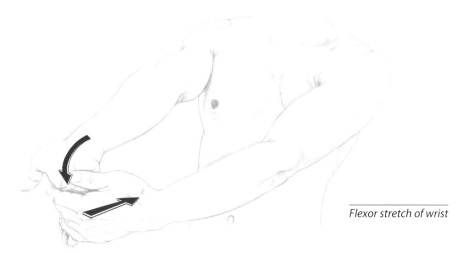

Flexor stretch of wrist

*Flexor stretch of the
hand and fingers*

Wrist Flexors – Stretch

1) Standing or seated. With your right elbow extended and your forearm supinated, place the fingers of your left hand across the palm of your right hand.

2) Using this point of contact on the hand, slowly extend the right wrist and digits (top image).

3) There are several variations of this stretch, including changing the point of contact to the middle or distal phalanges (bottom image).

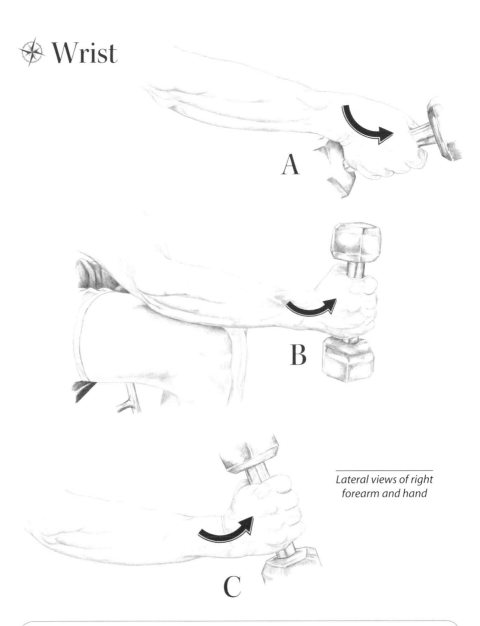

A

B

Lateral views of right forearm and hand

C

Wrist Abductors – Strengthen

1) Seated, with a dumbbell in your right hand. Rest your right forearm on your thigh so the dumbbell is out over your knee.

2) With your forearm in a neutral position (thumb toward the ceiling–A) and the wrist hanging in adduction, begin the exercise by slowly abducting your wrist (B).

3) When the wrist is fully abducted (C), return to the starting position.

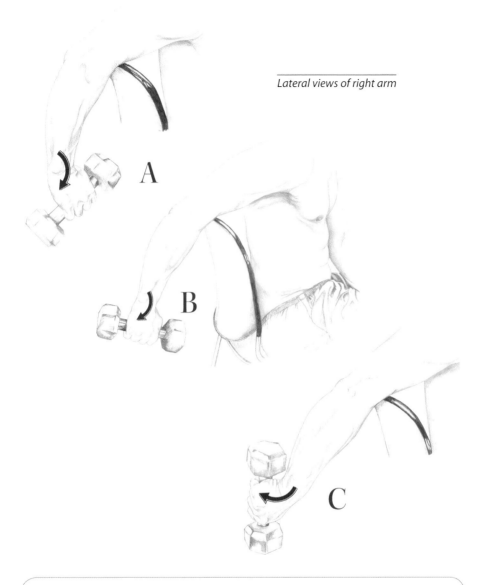

Lateral views of right arm

A

B

C

Wrist Adductors – Strengthen

1) Seated, with a dumbbell in your right hand. Put your right arm over the back of the chair (resting just above your inner elbow) and extend your elbow.

2) With your forearm in a neutral position (thumb pointed toward the chair–A), adduct your wrist by swinging the dumbbell away from the chair (B).

3) When the wrist is fully adducted (C), return to the starting position.

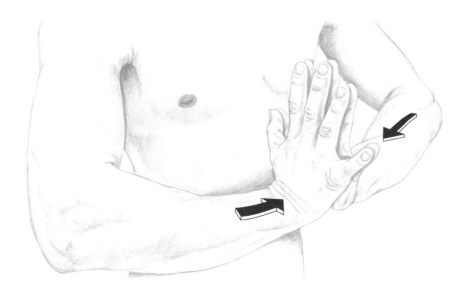

Finger Flexors – Stretch

1) Standing. Bring your palms together in front of your chest. Your forearms should be parallel with the floor and your fingers should be spread apart and pointing toward the ceiling.

2) As you gently press your palms together, slowly drop your wrists toward the floor.

✶ Vertebral Column

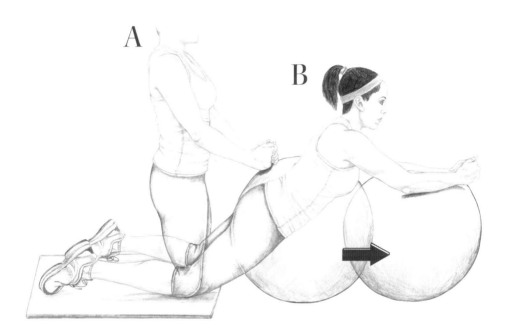

A

B

Vertebral Column Flexors – Strengthen

Variation 1 – On a big ball

1) Begin kneeling on a mat with a big ball in front of you. Interlace your fingers and set them on top of the ball (A).

2) Begin to slowly shift your weight forward. The ball will roll forward, changing your point of contact from your hands to your forearms to your elbows (B).

3) The objective here is to maintain a line of connection between your shoulders, hips and knees (thus working your abdominal muscles and other flexors).

4) Try to avoid "sticking your butt out" or collapsing your abdomen toward the floor. Also, lean forward only to a comfortable point and then pause for a deep breath. As you exhale, roll the ball back to your starting position.

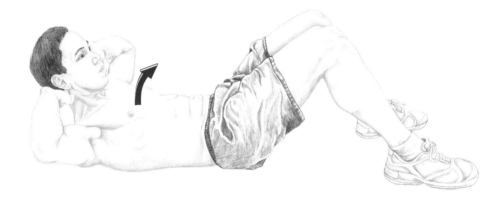

Vertebral Column Flexors – Strengthen

Variation 2 – On the floor

1) Supine, with your knees flexed and feet flat on the floor. Place both hands behind your head (or cross them in front of your chest).

2) As you exhale, slowly curl your head, neck and then thoracic spine up off the floor.

3) Keep in mind that you do not need to flex very far to engage the abdominals. Also, your hands should support the weight of your head but should not pull on your neck.

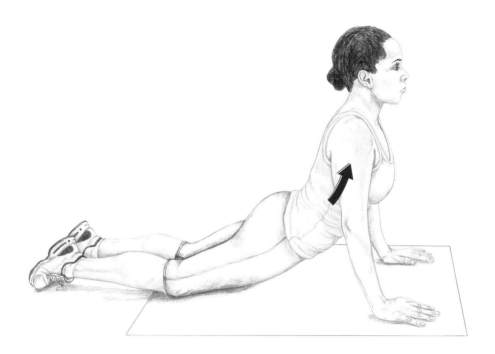

Vertebral Column Flexors – Stretch

Variation 1 – On the floor

1) Prone. Lying on your abdomen, set your palms on the floor at the level of your rIbs.

2) Slowly raise your upper torso, extending your spine and thorax. If possible, try to keep the anterior surface of your pelvis on the floor. If not, that's fine (as seen above).

✷ Vertebral Column

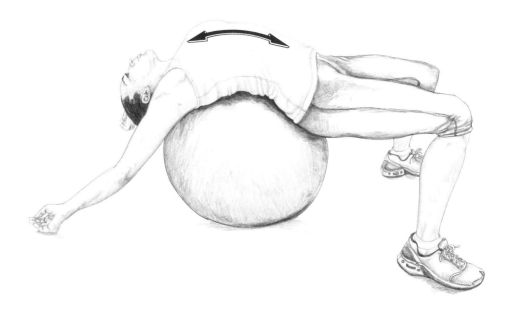

Vertebral Column Flexors – Stretch

Variation 2 – On a big ball

1) Begin sitting on a big ball. Roll your hips forward on the ball, allowing your spine to lay back on the ball in an extended position.

2) With the ball making contact with your lumbar and thoracic regions, set both feet flat on the floor for stability.

3) Take several deep breaths. To accentuate the stretch into the upper chest, bring your arms out to your sides.

4) To release from the stretch, slowly roll your spine forward off the ball, easing your spine up to an erect position.

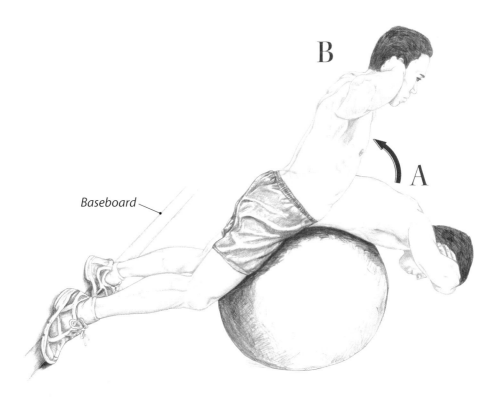

Baseboard

Vertebral Column Extensors – Strengthen

1) Prone on a big ball, next to a wall. Stabilize yourself by setting your feet against the baseboard and let your torso fold over the ball (A).

2) Set your hands behind your head (or in front of your chest) and, as you inhale, extend your torso (B). The front of your hips should press against the stationary ball.

3) Rise only to a comfortable point and then, exhaling, slowly return to the starting position.

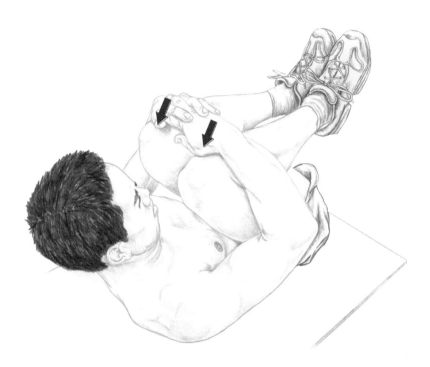

Vertebral Column Extensors – Stretch

Variation 1 – On the floor

1) Supine. Lying on your back, bring both of your knees up to your chest. Your head can either rest on the floor or slowly rise up toward your knees. Enjoy some nice, deep breaths.

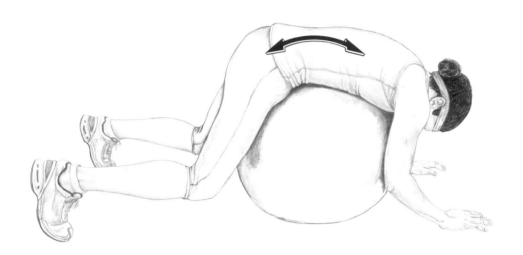

Vertebral Column Extensors – Stretch

Variation 2 – On a big ball

1) Begin kneeling in front of a big ball. Bring the ball in close and roll your torso over the top of it.

2) With the ball making contact with your chest, abdomen and part of your hips, be sure that both hands and feet are on the floor for stability.

3) Allow your head to passively flex down toward the floor.

✳ Vertebral Column

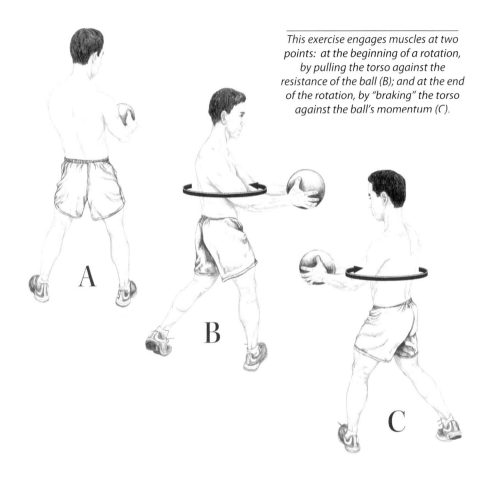

This exercise engages muscles at two points: at the beginning of a rotation, by pulling the torso against the resistance of the ball (B); and at the end of the rotation, by "braking" the torso against the ball's momentum (C).

A

B

C

Vertebral Column Rotators – Strengthen

Variation 1 – With a ball. Use caution not to torque your knees.

1) Standing, with a weighted ball in your hands (A).

2) With your feet set wider than your hips and the ball held away from your abdomen, begin to slowly rotate your torso to the right and then back to the left (B). When you have rotated all the way to the left, rotate back the right (C).

3) You can keep your heels planted or, to engage your hips, let them rise at the end of each twist. Use caution not to torque your knees at the end of each rotation.

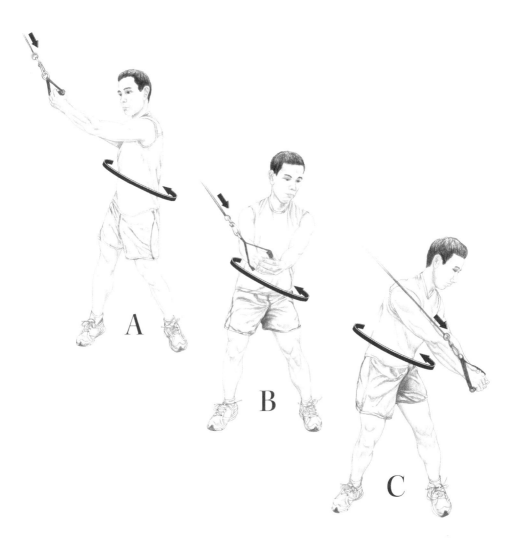

A

B

C

Vertebral Column Rotators – Strengthen

Variation 2 – With a pulley

1) Standing, with cable handle in both hands. The source of the cable resistance is at the ceiling level and over your right shoulder.

2) Begin with your torso and hips rotated a bit to the right (A). Then, as you rotate your torso to the left, bring the handle diagonally down and to the left (B, C).

3) Throughout the rotation, try to keep your elbows extended and your hands in front of your torso.

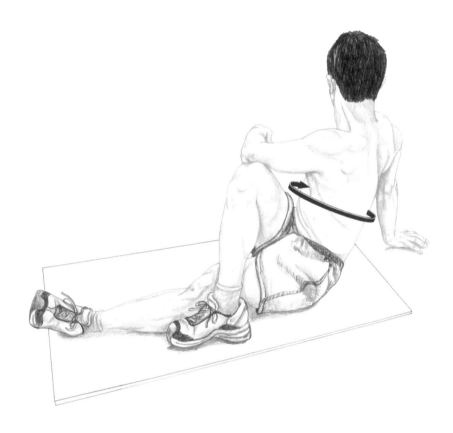

Vertebral Column Rotators – Stretch

Variation 1 – Leg crossed over

1) Sitting on the floor with your legs out in front of you. Cross your right foot over your left knee.

2) Set your left elbow on the outside of your right knee. Following your breath, slowly rotate your torso to the right.

3) As the stretch progresses, slide your right hand along the floor for stability. Also, rotating your head to the right will increase the intensity of the stretch. Be sure that your torso does not collapse as you rotate.

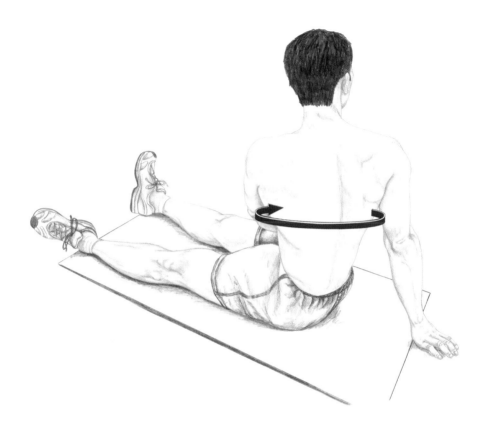

Vertebral Column Rotators – Stretch

Variation 2 – Legs out in front

1) Sitting on the floor with your legs out in front of you.

2) Set your right hand behind you and rotate your torso to the right. You can hook your left hand along the outside of your right thigh to stabilize the stretch.

3) Be sure that your torso does not collapse as you rotate.

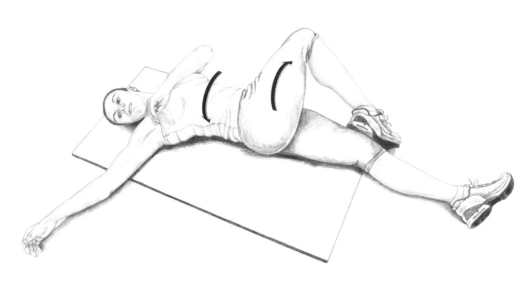

Vertebral Column Rotators – Stretch

Variation 3

1) Supine. Flex your right hip and knee. Rest your right foot on the outside of your left knee.

2) Use your left hand to gently bring your right knee across the body and over your left thigh. Your right hip will rise off of the floor.

3) To accentuate the stretch, reach your right hand out to the side and rotate your head to the right. A few deep breaths will feel nice.

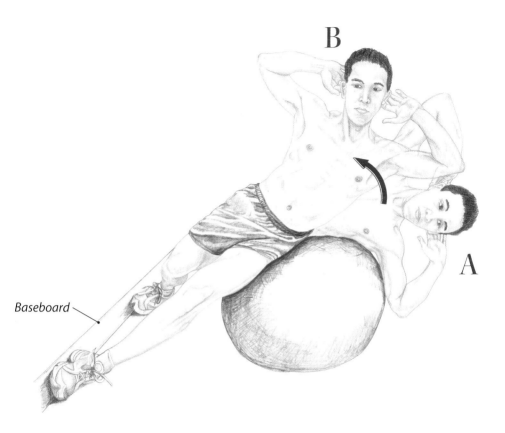

Baseboard

Vertebral Column Lateral Flexors – Strengthen

1) Set your left hip on a big ball. Shift your feet to the side and set them against the base of the wall, one foot in front of the other.

2) Adjust the ball and your hips so that your legs are at a 45-degree angle from the floor. Then curl the lateral side of your torso over the top of the ball. Now you are in position for the exercise (A).

3) With your fingers interlaced behind your head (or in front of your chest), laterally flex your torso (B). Rise only to a comfortable point and then slowly return to the starting position.

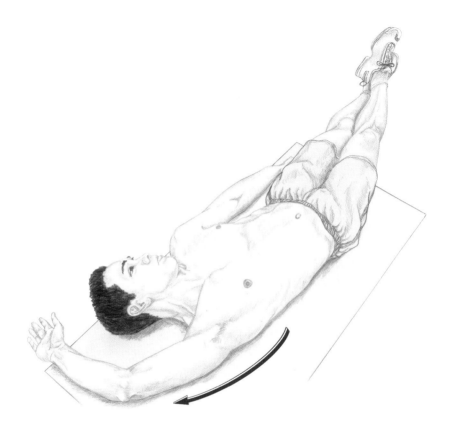

Vertebral Column Lateral Flexors – Stretch

Variation 1 – On the floor

1) Supine. Hook your right foot over your left ankle and reach your right arm up over your head.

2) Laterally flex your torso. Assist the stretch by reaching your left hand down toward your feet.

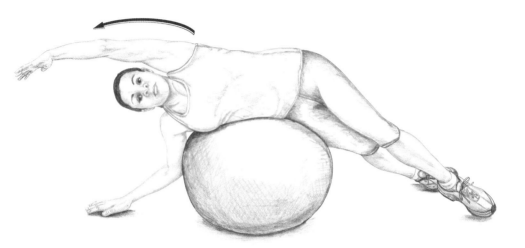

Vertebral Column Lateral Flexors – Stretch

Variation 2 – On a big ball

1) Begin kneeling beside a big ball. Leading with your right arm, slowly roll the right side of your torso over the top of the ball.

2) With the ball making contact with your rib cage and some of your hip, abduct your left arm over your head. For stability, be sure that your right hand and both feet are in contact with the floor.

3) To release from the stretch, reverse the process by rolling your right side off the ball.

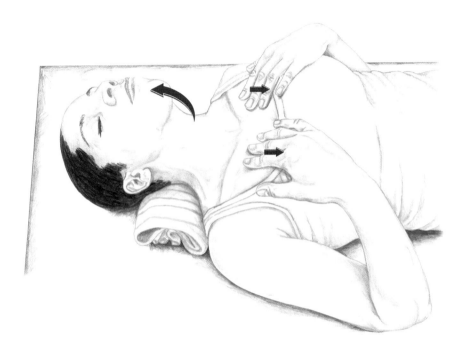

Neck Flexors – Stretch

1) Supine. Roll up a small towel and place it behind your neck. Then set both hands on your clavicles.

2) Without lifting your head, begin to extend your neck (leading with your chin). At the same time, use your fingers to gently pull the skin of the upper chest inferiorly.

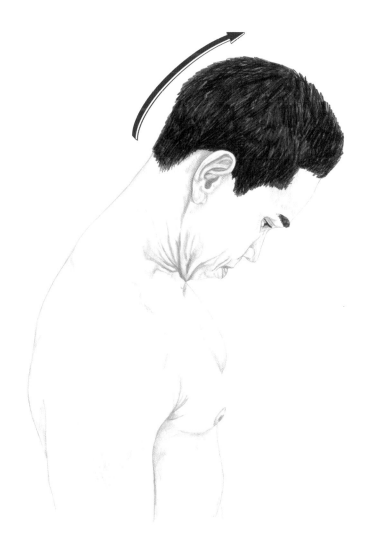

Neck Extensors – Stretch

1) Standing, with your arms at your sides. This stretch begins by tucking your chin, but much of the stretch comes from imagining the back of your head rising up and over your body.

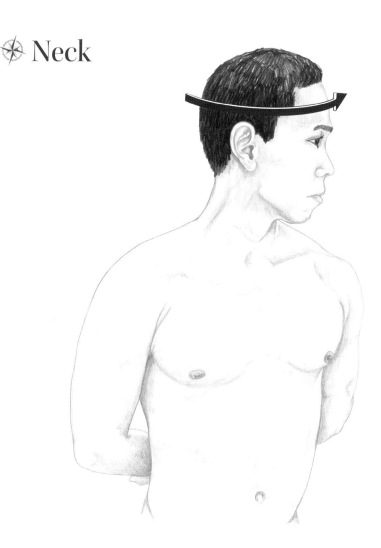

Neck Rotators – Stretch

1) Standing. With your arms behind your back (which will help stabilize the shoulders), rotate your head to the left.

2) Engaging your eyes by looking farther over your left shoulder will help to accentuate the stretch. Then ease out of the stretch and rotate your head to the right, stretching the opposite side.

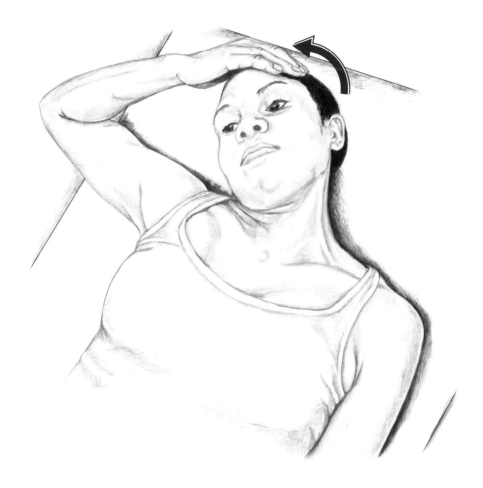

Neck Lateral Flexors – Stretch

1) Supine. Without lifting your head off of the floor or mat, laterally flex your head to the right.

2) Use your right hand to reach over your head for both support and a little more stretch.

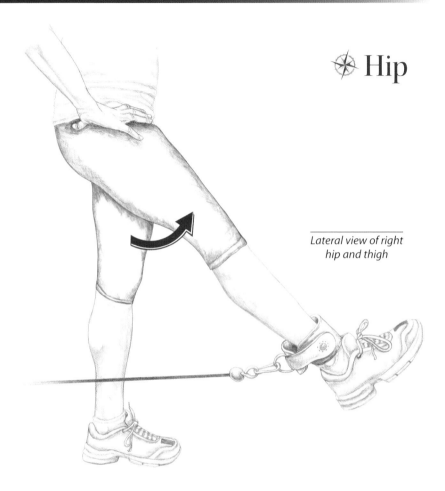

✳ Hip

*Lateral view of right
hip and thigh*

Hip Flexors – Strengthen

Variation 2 – With a pulley

1) Standing, with a cable strap around your right ankle. The source of the cable resistance is behind you and at floor level.

2) Stabilize yourself by holding onto the machine (or a wall).

3) Keeping your knee extended, slowly flex your right hip a comfortable distance and then return to the starting position.

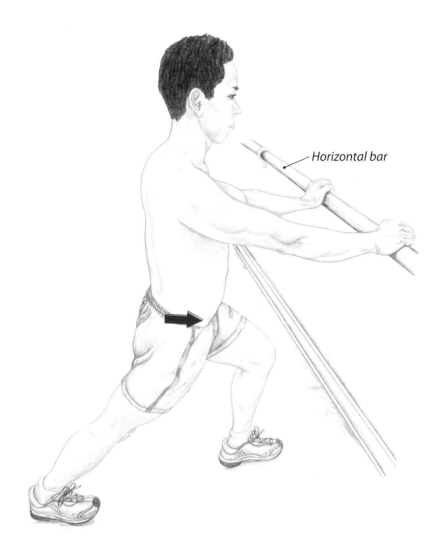

Horizontal bar

Hip Flexors – Stretch

1) Standing in front of a horizontal bar (or wall). Set both hands on the bar (about chest high) and bring your left foot forward and your right foot back.

2) Stabilizing with your arms, slowly shift your pelvis forward. Optimally, you will feel a stretch on the anterior surface of your right hip, as well as on your gastrocnemius and soleus muscles in your calf.

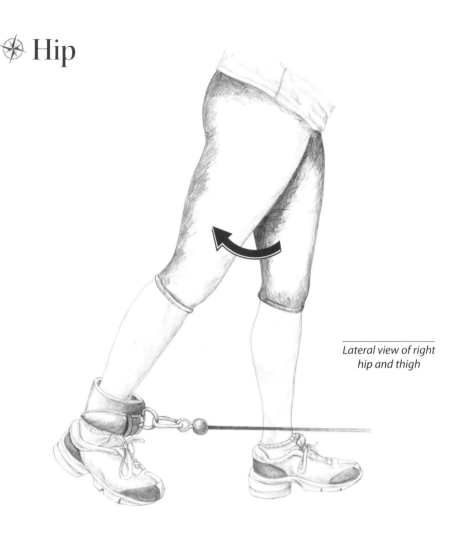

Lateral view of right hip and thigh

Hip Extensors – Strengthen

1) Standing, with a cable strap around your right ankle. The source of the cable resistance is in front of you and at floor level.

2) Stabilize yourself by holding onto the machine (or a wall) and slowly extend your right hip a comfortable distance. Then return to the starting position. During extension, be sure that your pelvis does not tilt anteriorly.

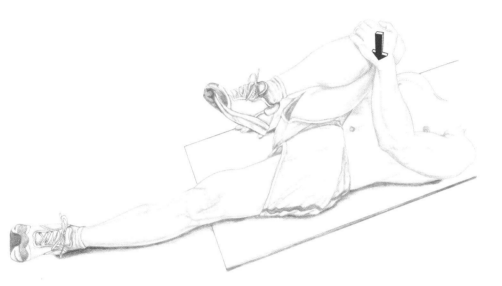

Anterior, lateral view

Hip Extensors – Stretch

Variation 1 – With your hands

1) Supine. Flex your right hip and knee, bringing your knee up toward your abdomen.

2) Cradle your knee with both hands and allow your left hip and thigh to remain in contact with the floor. Take several deep breaths.

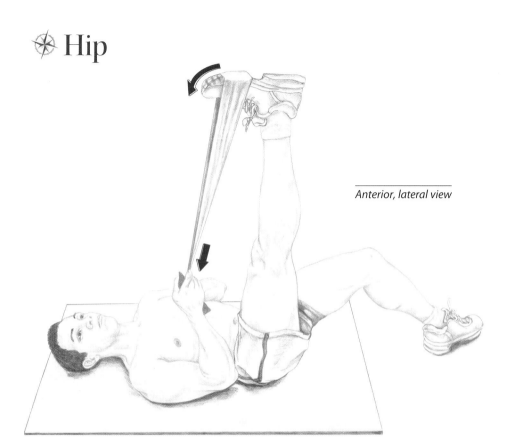

Anterior, lateral view

Hip Extensors – Stretch

Variation 2 – With a strap

1) Supine. Loop an elastic band (or towel) around the ball of your right foot.

2) With the thigh and leg on the floor and the band held with both hands, slowly begin to flex your right hip.

3) Assist the movement with the strap and be sure to keep your right knee extended. The left hip and knee can be slightly flexed (with the foot flat on the floor).

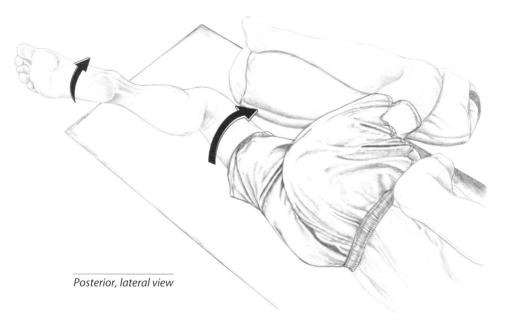

Posterior, lateral view

Hip Lateral Rotators – Strengthen

1) This exercise requires no weights, just lateral rotation of the hip against gravity. Lying on your right side, flex your left hip and knee and set a pillow underneath the knee for support.

2) Flex your right knee. Now you are ready for the exercise. Keeping your right knee on the floor, laterally rotate your right hip (swinging your right foot toward the ceiling). Do not allow your body to rotate.

3) Raise your foot only a comfortable distance and then return to the starting position.

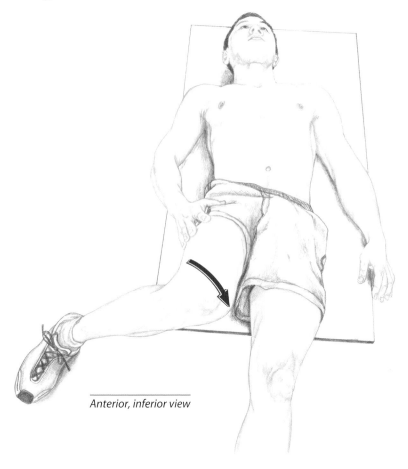

Anterior, inferior view

Hip Lateral Rotators – Stretch

1) Supine. Flex your right hip and knee to set your right foot at the level of your left knee. Then slowly walk out your foot laterally.

2) Following your breath, allow your right knee to slowly drop toward your left leg (internally rotating the hip). You can use your right hand on your thigh to gently deepen the stretch.

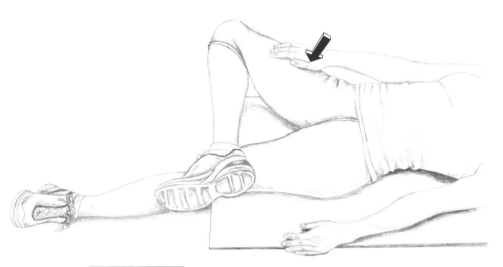

Anterior, lateral view

Hip Medial Rotators – Stretch

1) Supine. Cross your right foot above your left knee.

2) Following your breath, allow your right knee to slowly drop toward the floor. You can use your right hand to gently press your thigh toward the floor.

3) To prevent the right foot from sliding down the leg, you can loop a strap around your right ankle and hold it with your left hand.

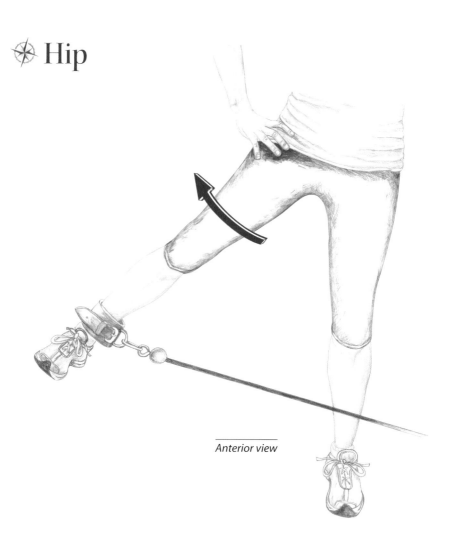

Anterior view

Hip Abductors – Strengthen

1) Standing, with a cable strap around your right ankle. The source of the cable resistance is from the side and at floor level.

2) Stabilize yourself by holding onto the machine (or a wall) and slowly abduct your right hip to a comfortable distance. Then return to the starting position. Be careful that your pelvis does not elevate as you abduct your hip.

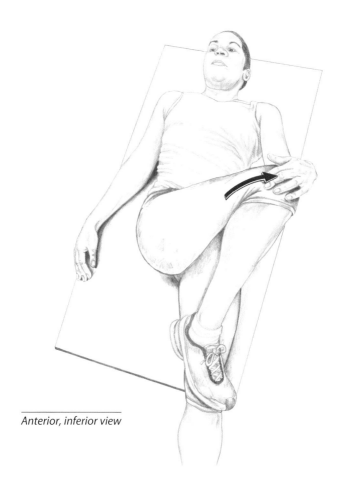

Anterior, inferior view

Hip Abductors – Stretch

Variation 1 – On the floor

1) Supine. Flex your right hip and knee, so that your thigh is flexed at 90 degrees.

2) Supporting your right knee with your left hand, slowly bring your knee across to the left.

3) Be sure that your right hip stays in contact with the floor (otherwise, this becomes a great low back stretch). A few deep breaths into the abdomen can help accentuate the stretch.

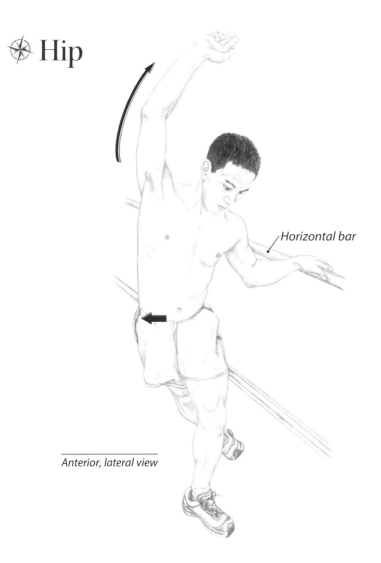

Horizontal bar

Anterior, lateral view

Hip Abductors – Stretch

Variation 2 – Standing

1) Standing next to a horizontal bar (or wall). Cross your right foot behind and to the left to your left foot.

2) Stabilizing with your left hand, abduct your right arm up and over your head. Finally, slowly lean your hips to your right. Optimally, you will feel a stretch on the lateral side of your right hip.

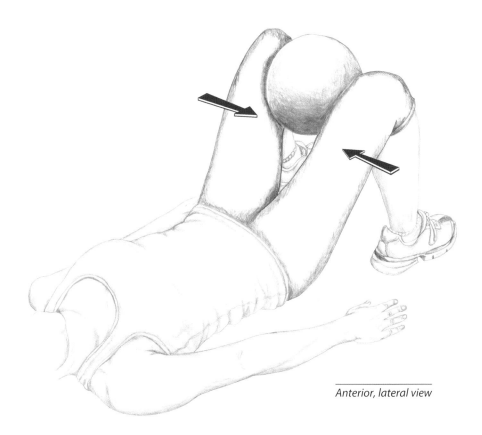

Anterior, lateral view

Hip Adductors – Strengthen

Variation 1 – On the floor

1) Supine. With your knees flexed and feet flat on the floor, place a small ball between your knees.

2) As you exhale, squeeze your knees together against the ball. As you inhale, relax your knees (but still hold the ball in place).

✳ Hip

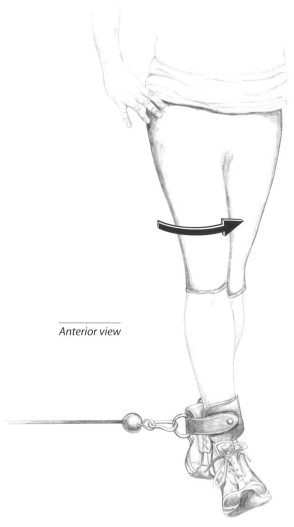

Anterior view

Hip Adductors – Strengthen

Variation 2 – With a pulley

1) Standing, with a cable strap around your right ankle. The source of the cable resistance is from the right side and at floor level.

2) Stabilize yourself by holding onto the machine (or wall). Slowly adduct your right hip by crossing your right foot in front of your left, and then slowly return to the starting position.

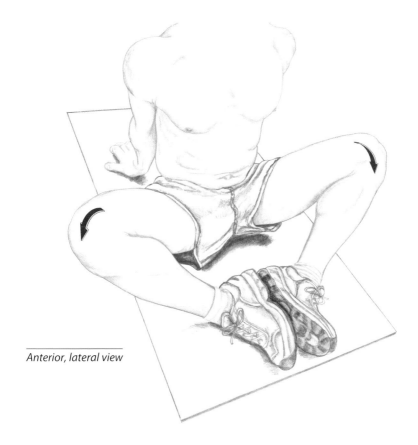

Anterior, lateral view

Hip Adductors – Stretch

1) Seated. Bring both feet together in front of you, sole to sole, and set both hands behind your hips for support.

2) Allow your knees to gently fall to the outside and begin to slowly press your pelvis anteriorly, stretching the adductors.

3) Maintaining a tall torso and taking deep breaths can accentuate the stretch.

4) To come out of the stretch, first release your torso and pelvis. Then roll back onto your spine and straighten your hips and knees.

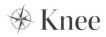 # ✳ Knee

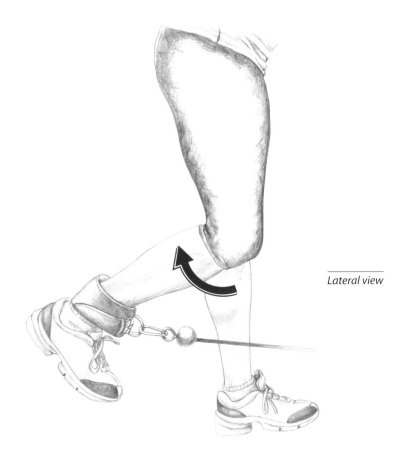

Lateral view

Knee Flexors – Strengthen

1) Standing, with a cable strap around your right ankle. The source of cable resistance is in front of you and at floor level.

2) Stabilize yourself by holding onto the machine (or a wall) and slowly flex your right knee. Flex the knee only to 90 degrees and be careful your pelvis does not tilt anteriorly.

3) Return to the starting position.

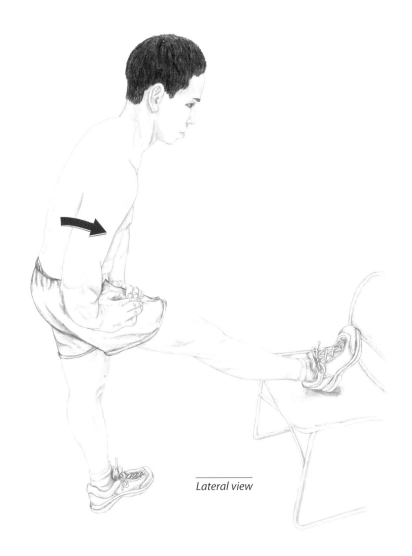

Lateral view

Knee Flexors – Stretch

Variation 1 – With a chair

1) Standing, with your right heel up on the seat of a chair.

2) With both hands on your right thigh and maintaining an erect spine, begin to slowly lean your torso forward.

3) As you feel a stretch along the back of your right thigh and knee, use your hands to insure that your hips do not begin to rotate to the left.

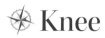

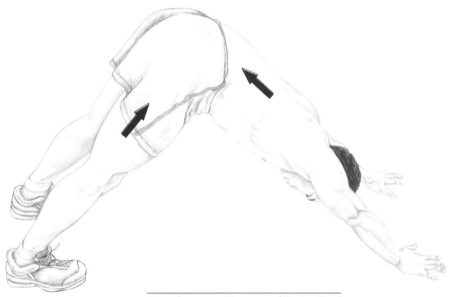

Better known as "Downward Facing Dog"
in yoga class, this is a fine stretch not only
for your knee flexors, but also for your
calves, hip extensors and low back.

Knee Flexors – Stretch

Variation 2 – On the floor

1) Begin on your hands and knees (hands beneath your shoulders, knees beneath your hips).

2) Curl your toes under your feet and push back on your hands. This will raise your hips and extend your knees.

3) Take several deep breaths and allow your neck to relax. It's all right if your heels do not touch the floor.

4) To come out of the stretch, flex your knees, bringing them to the floor, and uncurl your toes.

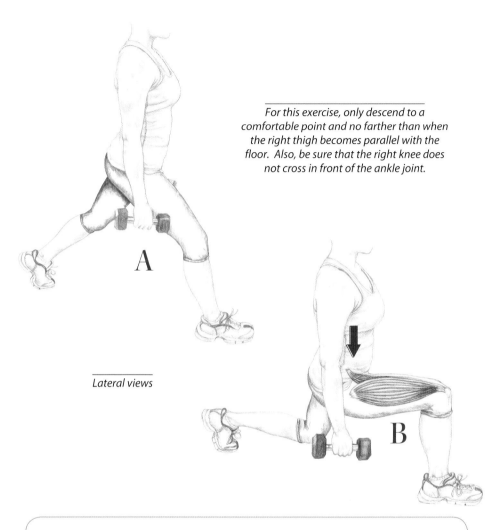

For this exercise, only descend to a comfortable point and no farther than when the right thigh becomes parallel with the floor. Also, be sure that the right knee does not cross in front of the ankle joint.

A

Lateral views

B

Knee Extensors – Strengthen

1) Standing, with a dumbbell in each hand. Step your right foot forward and your left foot back (A).

2) Maintaining an erect torso, slowly drop your hips and left knee down toward the floor (B). Your right hip and knee will flex with this action.

3) Slowly raise your hips back to the starting position. For the other side, step your left foot forward.

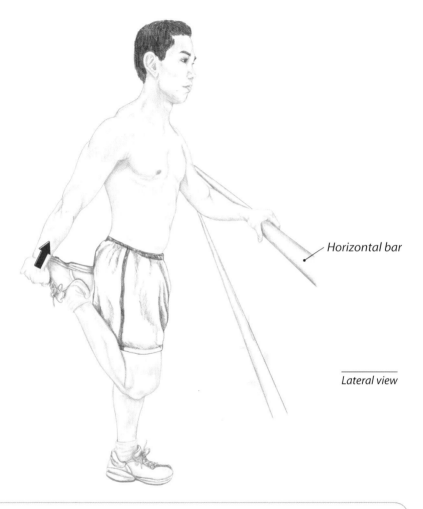

Horizontal bar

Lateral view

Knee Extensors – Stretch

1) Standing in front of a horizontal bar (or wall). Stabilize yourself with your left hand.

2) Flex your right knee. As you do, reach down with your right hand and grasp the top of your right foot.

3) Maintaining an erect torso and, without tilting the pelvis anteriorly, use your hand to slowly raise your foot (further flexing the knee).

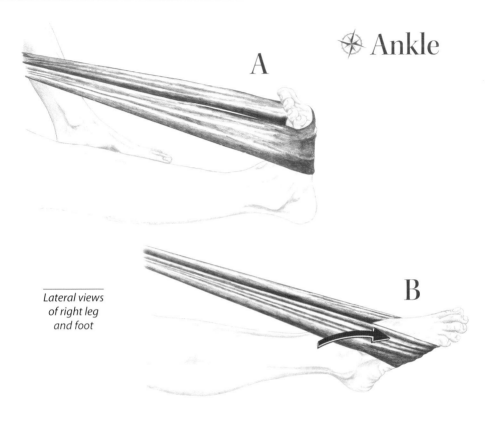

�֎ Ankle

A

B

*Lateral views
of right leg
and foot*

Ankle Plantar Flexors – Strengthen

Variation 1 – With a strap

1) Sitting on the floor, with your legs out in front of you. Loop an elastic strap around the ball of your right foot.

2) Pull the ends of the strap so your ankle is dorsiflexed (A). Then slowly plantar flex your ankle against the strap's resistance (B).

3) When the ankle is fully plantar flexed, slowly return to the starting position. (If the strap slips off your foot, you can loop it once around the ball of your foot for greater stability.)

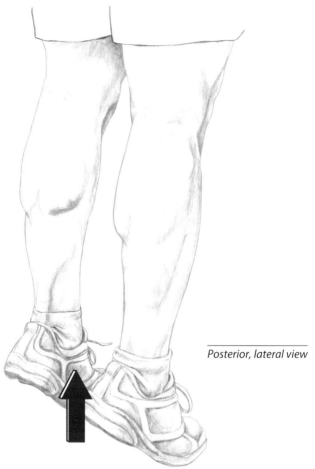

Posterior, lateral view

Ankle Plantar Flexors – Strengthen

Variation 2 – Standing

1) Standing next to a chair (or a wall). Holding the back of the chair for stability, set your feet hip-width apart.

2) Lifting your body weight, raise your heels (plantar flexing your ankles).

3) Slowly lower your heels and return to the starting position.

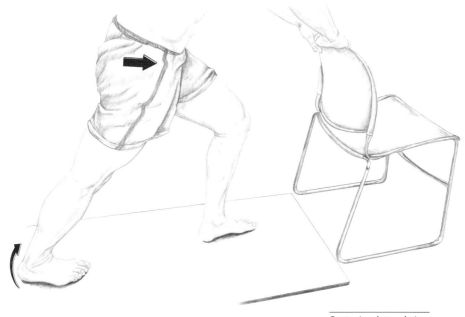

Posterior, lateral view

Ankle Plantar Flexors – Stretch

1) Standing behind a chair (or next to a wall). Set both hands on the back of the chair and slide your right foot back.

2) Keeping the heel of your right foot on the floor, slowly shift your hips forward, moving your weight onto your left foot and hands.

3) To stretch the soleus specifically, perform the same stretch with the knee slightly flexed.

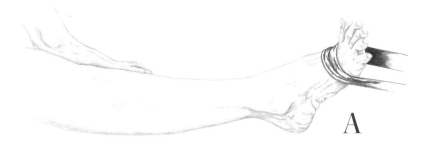

Lateral views of right leg and foot

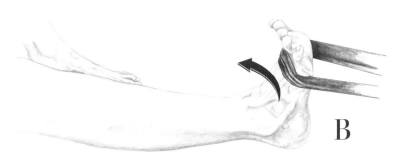

Ankle Dorsiflexors – Strengthen

This exercise is best performed with a partner.

1) Sitting on the floor with your legs out in front of you. Loop an elastic strap around the top of your right foot.

2) Have your partner sit in front of you and hold the ends of the strap. With your partner providing moderate tension, begin with your ankle plantar flexed (A).

3) Slowly dorsiflex your ankle against the strap's resistance (B). Slowly return to the starting position.

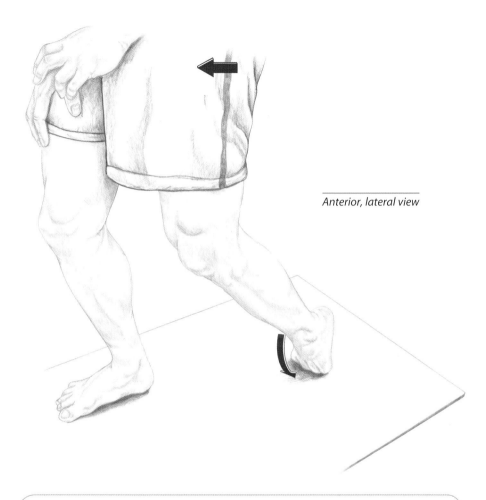

Anterior, lateral view

Ankle Dorsiflexors – Stretch

1) Standing. Shift your left foot back. (You can stabilize yourself by setting your hands on a chair or wall.)

2) Roll your toes over so that the top of your foot is against the floor. Then lean your weight forward, gently bringing the front of your ankle toward the floor.

3) Shifting the direction of the stretch (laterally or medially) can help to expand the scope of the stretch.

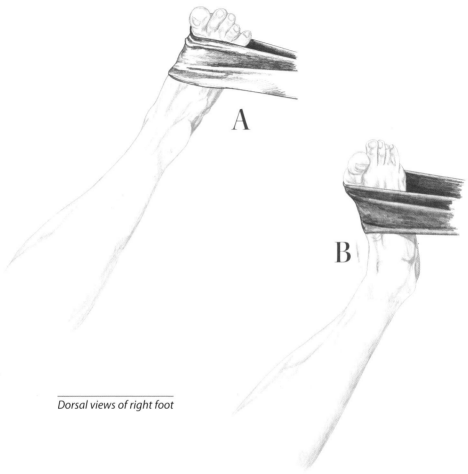

Dorsal views of right foot

Foot Invertors – Strengthen

This exercise is best performed with a partner.

1) Sitting on the floor with your legs out in front of you. Loop an elastic strap around the inside of your right foot.
2) Have your partner sit to your right, holding the ends of the strap with moderate tension. Begin with your foot everted (A).
3) Slowly invert your foot against the strap's resistance (B).
4) When the foot is fully inverted, slowly return to the starting position.

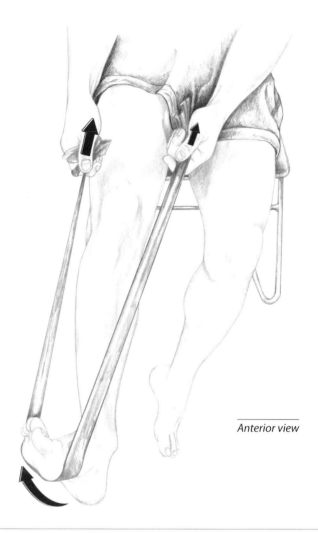

Anterior view

Foot Invertors – Stretch

1) Seated. Loop an elastic strap (or towel) around the arch of your right foot.

2) Extend your right knee and dorsiflex your right ankle. Then, using the strap to "steer" the sole of the foot, passively evert your foot.

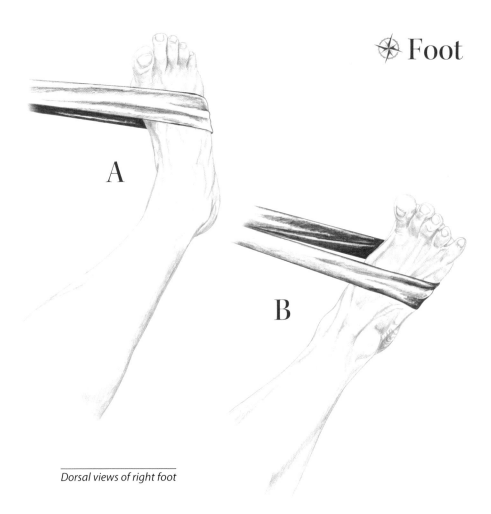

A

B

Dorsal views of right foot

Foot Evertors – Strengthen

This exercise is best performed with a partner.

1) Sitting on the floor with your legs out in front of you. Loop an elastic strap around the outside of your right foot.

2) Have your partner sit to your left, holding the ends of the strap with moderate tension. Begin with your foot inverted (A).

3) Slowly evert your foot against the strap's resistance (B). When the foot is fully everted, slowly return to the starting position.

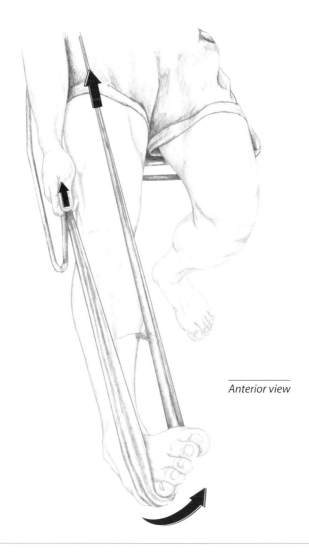

Anterior view

Foot Evertors – Stretch

1) Seated. Loop an elastic strap (or towel) around the ball of your right foot. Extend your right knee and plantar flex your right ankle.

2) Using the strap to "steer" the sole of the foot, invert the foot.

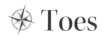

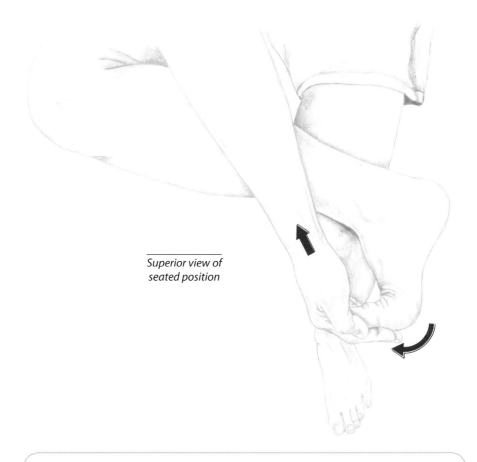

Superior view of
seated position

Toe Flexors – Stretch

1) Seated, with your right foot on your left knee.
2) Passively extend the toes of your right foot with your right hand.

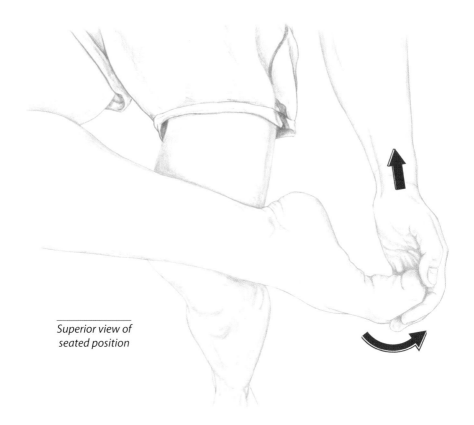

Superior view of seated position

Toe Extensors – Stretch

1) Seated, with your right foot on your left knee.
2) Passively flex the toes of your right foot with your left hand.

Index